USMLE STEP 2 CK PEARLS
Over 500 High Yield Facts To Ace The Exam

John Thomas, MD

Copyright © 2020 John Thomas

All rights reserved. This book or any portion thereof may not be reproduced or used in any manner whatsoever without the express written permission of the publisher.

First Edition: July 2020

Disclaimer: This book does not in any way establish or recommend any clinical guidelines or medical practice. The information presented in this book is solely intended to be used for test preparation and not for treating patients. I take no responsibility for any errors you may make using the information presented in this book.

The author is not affiliated in any way with the United States Medical Licensing Exam.

PREFACE

This slim book is designed to be a concise review of the most essential, aka, "high yield", facts necessary for success on the United States Medical Licensing Exam Step 2 CK. The book is also relevant for USMLE Step 3. Hundreds of sources, both primary and secondary, were consulted while writing this book and only the most relevant facts were selected for inclusion. Note that I purposely avoided categorizing the facts by specialty, and the facts are presented in a random order. This is on purpose because on test day you will not be tested in blocks by subject matter. This book is designed to be a "cross-trainer" and force you to think like you would on test day. The knowledge presented is in multiple formats throughout the book: as statement of fact, clinical correlation, or question. Certain concepts are repeated as they are either difficult concepts or of greater importance such that I wanted to emphasize them. Use this as a final review *after* you have conducted your primary study. I advise on using it during your final three weeks of study and thoroughly memorizing the facts presented.

I have written this book in an abbreviated format in a colloquial voice that is designed for quick consumption. Therefore, I have eliminated full sentences as much as possible. Please make sure to read the list of abbreviations before reading the book.

Lastly, this book arose at the request of a small group of medical students that I had tutored. The facts presented here were workshopped over the course of a year during the tutoring sessions and perfected for maximal retention. If you received a copy of this book from a source other than the Amazon.com store, please purchase a copy from Amazon.com as that is the only authorized seller. I am not a practicing physician, but an independent medical researcher. I tutor medical students and I write about nutrition. Thus, sales from this book are a significant source of my income that allows me to support my family. Thank You.

TESTIMONIALS

"Dr. Thomas, I was looking for a very high score on Step 2 CK to make up for my average Step 1 score. I could not get that last boost I needed until I read your book. After using the tips in your book I was able to shoot my score into the 250's. Thanks." – Paul O., New York, NY USA

"Sir, I went from a fail to passing CK by 20 points on my second attempt after using the pearls presented in your book. Thank you from the bottom of my heart as I am now eligible to apply for residency." – Kashif K., Karachi, Pakistan

"Your book was concise and to the point. It didn't waste my time. I was able to use it to comfortably pass the exam." – Bryan D., Miami, FL USA

"Great book for last minute review. I used it just before I gave the exam to refresh all the topics I had studied. I was super happy when I saw my exam results!" – Arjun P., New Delhi, India

ABBREVIATIONS

abx - antibiotics
ams – altered mental status
cc – clinical correlation. (a short clinical vignette)
dx – diagnosis
ddx – differential diagnosis
h/o – history of
mcc – most common cause
moa – method of action
n/v – nausea and vomiting
pe – physical exam
ppx - prophylaxis
pt – patient
pts – patients
rx – treatment
se – side effect
yo – year old

USMLE STEP 2 CK PEARLS

1. Aldosterone gets rid off acid from the body. So, increasing aldosterone leads to metabolic alkalosis and decreasing aldosterone (as in 21-hydroxylase deficiency) leads to metabolic acidosis.

2. Dopamine ("good" for a man) inhibits Prolactin (not "good" for a man). Prolactin inhibits Leutenizing Hormone, which leads to making more testosterone.

3. Vibrio vulnificus linked to diarrhea in patients with liver disease who consume contaminated shellfish. There is also an increased incidence of developing bullous skin lesions.

4. Diarrhea (non bloody) + flushing + wheezing + eat *fresh fish* → Scombroid, which is histamine fish poisoning.

5. Sideroblastic anemia associated with alcoholism, INH, and myelodysplasia. The <u>only</u> anemia associated with increased iron!! Diagnosis ("dx"): Prussian blue stain. There is no therapy.

6. Vitamin B12 deficiency vs. Folate deficiency

Vit B12 deficiency	Folate deficiency
Neurological abnormalities	---
Peripheral neuropathy	---
Increased homocysteine	Increased homocysteine
Increased methylmalonic acid	----

7. Parvovirus B19 invades the bone marrow and freezes the growth of precursor cells in the marrow, therefore the reticulocyte count is abnormally low. Really bad for a sickle cell pt.

8. **Hemolytic Uremic Syndrome (HUS)** is the "triad" of symptoms = hemolytic anemia + thrombocytopenia + uremia. Will see increased creatinine. **Thrombotic Thrombocytopenic Purpura (TTP)** is the "pentad" of symptoms = HUS + fever + CNS abnormalities.

9. CHF treatments by NYHA Class. *Don't use CCB to rx systolic CHF!*

NYHA Class	Treatment
I	(a) ACE-I/ARB + Beta Blocker (older). (b) Valsartan + Sacubitril (newer). (c) Ivabradine.
II	Furosemide (lasix)
III	Spironolactone or Bidil
IV	Milrinone or Dobutamine

10. Age related macular degeneration (ARMD) -central vision lost, peripheral vision intact.
    Dry type → central loss of vision, multiple drusen. Takes years. No cure or rx.
    Wet type → Straight line appears wavy or curved. Sudden loss of vision. Rx is VEGF inhibitors ranibizumab, pegaptanib.

11. The 4 P's that cause Pleuritic chest pain: Pericarditis (pain gets better sitting upright and leaning forward), Pleural Effusion, Pulmonary Embolism, and Pancreatitis (severe epigastric abdominal pain that radiates to the back with relief by leaning forward).

12. Bilateral infiltrates on CXR seen in: CHF, ARDS, and PCP Pneumonia ("bilateral fluffy infiltrates")

13. Crackles ("Rales") can be heard in either Pneumonia (focal consolidations in lungs) or in Pulmonary Edema (worse at the base of the lungs and bilateral). Pulmonary Edema can lead to CHF, ARDS, and PCP pneumonia.

14. In PCP pneumonia, LDH levels are always increasing

15. MI Differentials (retrosternal chest pain)
    a. Esophageal Spasm – But, relieved by nitrates so not MI
    b. GERD

16. Piperacillin/Tazobactam, Cefepime, Carbapenems (Imipenem, Meropenem, Ertapenem):
    a. Pseudomonas
    b. Neutropenic fever
    c. Renal abscess

17. Rheumatoid Arthritis vs. Osteoarthritis

RA	OA
Bilateral	Unilateral
Better with use	Worse with use
MCP, PIP affected	PIP, DIP affected (same in
	Psoriatic arthritis)

    Remember the joints of the hand with "*M*innesota *P*olice *D*epartment"
    a. *M*CP = Knuckles
    b. *P*IP (Bouchard's Nodules) = Middle joints
    c. *D*IP (Heberden's Nodules) = Joints closest to finger tip

18. Differentials for non-cardiogenic pulmonary edema (PCWP<12)
    a. ARDS
    b. Aspirin overdose

19. Jaundice differentials
    a. Choledocholithiasis – painful jaundice
    b. Cholangitis – painful jaundice (c-h are painless jaundice)

  c. Primary Biliary Cirrhosis
  d. Hemochromatosis
  e. Alpha-1-Antitrypsin Deficiency
  f. Cancer
  g. Stricture
  h. Wilson's Disease

20. "**U** **G**o **C**razy, **C** Dr. **R**ogers"
  a. **U**nconjugated Bilirubinemia : **G**ilbert and **C**rigler
  b. **C**onjugated Bilirubinemia : **D**ubin and **R**otor

21. Lower GI bleeding differentials
  a. Painless bright red blood per rectum (brbpr) = diverticular hemorrhage (diverticulosis)
  b. Painful brbpr = ischemic colitis (watershed area doesn't get enough O2 leading to hypotension). Shows up on CT. Rx: Bowel rest. cc: old guy will get shock, look for dehydration, bloody diarrhea + abdominal pain.
  c. Painful with no bleeding = diverticulitis

22. Pain associated with eating food differentials
  a. Pain while eating food = gastroparesis, gastric ulcer
  b. Pain after eating = duodenal ulcer, mesenteric (chronic) ischemia. For mesenteric ischemia look for acute pain out of proportion to physical exam. Risk factors: atherosclerosis, AFib, cocaine use. Dx: arteriography, doesn't show up on CT or Xray. Rx: Revascularization.

23. Feels like an MI, but EKG is negative. Rx for both is CCB, Nitrates
  a. Prinzmetal's angina
  b. Esophageal spasm

24. Rx for diverticulitis and cholecystitis: NPO diet + IV fluids + IV antibiotics
  Rx for pancreatitis: NPO diet + IV fluids

25. Metoclopramide side effects: hyperprolactinemia, tardive dyskinesia (rare)

26. Hyperviscosity syndrome (headache, blurry vision, tinnitus, HTN, splenomegaly, thrombosis) is seen in:
  a. Polycythemia Vera
  b. Chronic Lymphocytic Leukemia (CLL)
  c. Waldenstrom Macroglobulinemia

27. ITP (Idiopathic Thrombocytopenia Purpura) and Warm AIHA have the same Rx:
  a. Prednisone
  b. IV IgG to raise platelets quickly in acute cases
  c. Splenectomy for refractory cases
  d. Rituximab

28. Myelodysplastic Syndrome (MDS)
    a. Asymptomatic pancytopenia despite hypercellular bone marrow
    b. Dx: 5q deletion, sideroblasts, Increased MCV, Pelger-Huet anomaly
    c. Rx: Transfusion as needed, EPO, Azacitidine, Lenalidomide if 5q deletion

29. Myelofibrosis
    a. Pancytopenia + Bone marrow fibrosis (leading to enlarged liver and spleen)
    b. Dx: Tear-drop shaped cells
    c. Rx: Thalidomide (increases bone marrow production), Ruxolitinib (inhibits JAK2)

30. Rx for ITP (Idiopathic/Immune Thrombocytopenic Purpura)
    a. Steroids (if platelets < 30k)
    b. IV IgG (if platelets < 10k) + Anti-Rho (if pt. is Rh+) + Platelet transfusion (if active bleeding)
    c. Splenectomy or Rituximab (anti-CD20)
    d. If Splenectomy did not work
        i. Romiplostim or Eltrombopag [These are platelet receptor modifiers]
        ii. Azathioprine / Cyclosporine /Mycophenolate

31. Rx for Hairy Cell Leukemia
    a. Cladribine or Pentostatin

32. Rx for Aplastic Anemia
    a. Antithymocyte globulin and either cyclosporine or tacrolimus
    b. Alemtuzumab – anti-CD52 agent that suppresses T cells

33. Newest add on Rx for NYHA Class I CHF?
    a. Valsartan (ARB) + Sacubitril (nephrolysin inhibitor)
    b. Ivabradine (Calcium funny channel inhibitor)

34. Add on Rx for SLE → Belimumab (doesn't work in blacks though)

35. Pegvisomant → GH receptor antagonist at the liver, blocks production of IGF-1. Used in the rx of acromegaly

36. OCP (estrogen) associated diseases
    a. Porphyria Cutanea Tarda – deficiency in uroporphyrinogen decarboxylase. Symptoms: onycholysis, skin blisters, hypertrichosis, tea-colored urine. Differential: Acute Intermittent Porphyria – not estrogen associated. Will see *psychiatric* symptoms.
    b. Benign Intracranial HTN (pseudotumor cerebri). Rx: Acetazolamide, VP shunt

37. Calcium Channel Blockers (CCB)
    a. For HTN Rx: Amlodipine (also to expel kidney stones < 7mm), Felodipine
    b. For rate control Rx as in AFib: Diltiazem, Verapamil

38. Rotary Nystagmus causes
    a. Benign paroxysmal positional vertigo (bppv) → Dx with rotary nystagmus on Dix-Hallpike maneuver
    b. PCP intoxication

39. Hepatopulmonary (liver-lung) Syndrome Triad
    a. Cirrhosis
    b. Hypoxia
    c. Orthodeoxia aka Platypnea – worse SOB on sitting upright from a horizontal position
    Will see increased A-a gradient. Dx: Contrast echo or T99 labeled albumin perfusion study.

40. cc: Pain in hand and radial side of wrist. Occurs when she is gripping objects and squeezing things. Finkelstein test (grasp the thumb and ulnar deviate the hand) is abnormal. This is De Quervain Tenosynovitis. Rx: NSAID and splinting

41. Optic Neuritis (seen in Multiple Sclerosis, Encephalitis, Lupus). Rx: steroids
    a. Unilateral loss of vision in 1-2 weeks
    b. Swelling of the optic disc
    c. Diminished perception of red colors
    d. Marcus-Gunn pupil – pupil constricts only when light is shown in unaffected eye

42. Cavernous Sinus Thrombosis = Mucormycosis
    a. Double vision, headache, sinusitis, extraocular movements impaired, proptosis, ptosis, chemosis (red and swollen conjunctiva)

43. Di George Syndrome = Thymic hypoplasia = T cells *absent*
    a. Cardiac and facial defects
    b. Hypocalcemia due to defect/absent parathyroid glands
    c. Rx: Bone marrow transplant

44. Down Syndrome
    a. Duodenal atresia → bilious vomiting, double bubble sign, polyhydramnios
    b. VSD
    c. TOF
    d. Quad screen: Decreased: *AFP, UE3*. Increased: *Beta-HCG, Inhibin A* (Same lab results seen in Turner Syndrome)
        i. Ddx: Edwards (18) → Everything is low
        ii. Ddx: Patau (13) → Everything is normal except AFP is increased. ("AFPatau is high")

45. Maternal cocaine use in pregnancy can lead to:
    a. Coarctation of the aorta

    b. Intestinal atresia → bilious vomiting, double bubble sign, multiple air fluid levels. (smoking in pregnancy can also lead to intestinal atresia)

46. Long QT Syndrome (Lange Jervell Nielsen Syndrome)
    a. Hearing loss from birth
    b. Syncope
    c. Family history of sudden cardiac death (from torsades de pointes)
    d. Normal vitals and pe

47. Charcot-Marie-Tooth disease
    a. Cc: 12 yo child w/ progressive leg weakness, high arched foot (pes cavus), hammer toes, "champagne-bottle legs"
    b. This is a hereditary motor and sensory neuropathy of the peripheral nervous system whose pathophysiology and treatment are still not well understood.
    c. Peroneal muscle atrophy → foot drop
    d. Vibratory sense and general sense lost in a glove and stocking pattern
    e. Dx: nerve conduction studies
    f. Rx: physical therapy

48. Most common heart sounds to know cold!
    a. PDA, Mitral Regurgitation, Aortic Stenosis

49. Never use a calcium channel blocker (CCB) with pulmonary edema because it can lead to peripheral edema and pitting edema.

50. Leukocyte Adhesion Deficiency = adhesion defect in neutrophils. Cc: massive leukocytosis and high fever, delayed separation of the umbilical cord

51. Angioedema → C1esterase deficiency → Increased C1 complement

52. Know your DSM-5 psych terminology differentials. Ex: Baby blues vs. post-partum depression

53. You see buzzword "yellow-green discharge" in the context of STD's think trichomoniasis

54. Cervical Motion Tenderness differentials (Chlamydia and Gonorrhea are the #1 cause for all 3 diseases).
    a. No fever, no abdominal pain → *Cervicitis*
    b. Fever, Abdominal Pain, Elevated wbc
        i. Abdominal pain present → *Tubo-Ovarian Abscess*
        ii. No abdominal pain → *PID* (pelvic inflammatory disease)56

55. Cc: A 61 yo healthcare worker has had many vaccines recently, but what vaccine specific to his field of work does he need?
    a. Hepatitis B vaccine

56. Paraneoplastic Syndromes
    a. Renal Cell Carcinoma → EPO → Polycythemia
    b. Squamous Cell Carcinoma → PTH-rp → Hypercalcemia
    c. Small Cell Cancer → ACTH → Cushing Syndrome
        i. Small Cell Cancer → ADH → SIADH
    d. Adenocarcinoma → Hypertrophic osteodystrophy (Bamberger-Marie Syndrome) – wrist pain, ankle pain, clubbing of fingers

57. Cc: Woman with pelvic pain several days *before her period* and continues until period ends?
    a. Dx: U/S or MRI – initial test. Laparoscopy – best test
    b. Rx: 1st line – OCP, Danazol (androgen), Leuprolide (GnRH agonist)

58. Retinal Artery Occlusion vs. Retinal Vein Occlusion

	Retinal Artery Occlusion	Retinal Vein Occlusion
Appearance:	Pale Retina + Dark Macula ("Cherry red macula)	Extravasation of blood into retina ("tortuous appearance")
Rx:	100% O2, Acetazolamide, Thrombolytics	Ranibizumab

59. Meningitis = fever, headache, photophobia, stiff neck

60. Staph aureus is the mcc of bacterial meningitis (*neutrophilic* predominance) after recent neurosurgery.

61. Listeria is the mcc of meningitis in immunocompromised, elderly, neonates, and alcoholics.

62. Cryptococcus (fungal meningitis) → meningitis in HIV pt. with very low CD4 (<50). Increased lymphocytes, decreased glucose.

63. Cc: Old man with pneumonia + fever + bilateral interstitial infiltrates + cough + diarrhea + AMS + *hyponatremia* → Legionella. Rx: Moxifloxacin

64. Cc: HIV pt. with CD4<50, *blurry vision* → CMV retinitis. Dx: direct retinal visualization. Rx: Ganciclovir or Valganciclovir

65. Young female smoker at risk for
    a. Prinzmetal angina/variant angina – transient ST elevation. Rx: Nifedipine (CCB)
    b. Raynaud's phenomenon
    c. Migraine headaches
    d. DVT/Pulmonary Embolism

66. Rash on palms & soles seen in
    a. Secondary syphilis

    b. Erythema multiforme – targetoid, post HSV or Mycoplasma, drug reaction
    c. Toxic shock syndrome – tampon use often a cause
    d. Porphyria cutanea tarda – rash on dorsum of hands

67. Plasmapheresis vs. Exchange Transfusion
    a. Plasmapheresis – TTP, HUS, Autoimmune disease, Goodpasture syndrome
    b. ET – Sickle Cell Disease, Newborn jaundice w/ total bilirubin >20

68. Premature birth concerns (baby at risk for the following)
    a. Brain – intraventricular hemorrhage
    b. Lungs – prematurity of lungs (hypoplasia) → surfactant deficiency → ARDS
    c. Eye – retinopathy
    d. Intestines - necrotizing enterocolitis
    e. Nutrition – iron deficiency anemia

69. Elevated Beta-HCG occurs in
    a. Ectopic pregnancy
    b. Molar pregnancy
    c. Choriocarcinoma
    d. Seminoma (normal alpha-fetoprotein)
    e. Mixed germ cell tumor

70. Widened Mediastinum
    a. Aortic dissection
    b. Boerhaave Syndrome
    c. Acute mediastinitis (post-surgery complication, will see puss in the mediastinum)
    d. Necrotizing mediastinitis (complication of retropharyngeal abscess)

71. Must be sure pt. does not have Hep B or Hep C before Rituximab can be used

72. Cancers that metastasize to the bones think "lead kettle" / PBKTL
    a. Prostate – blastic
    b. Breast – mixed
    c. Kidney – lytic
    d. Thyroid – lytic
    e. Lungs – lytic

73. Abnormal ristocetin assay (tests platelet adhesion to endothelial lining)
    a. vWD
    b. Bernard-Soulier (decreased platelet count possible)

74. Digoxin has never been proven to lower mortality in CHF! Don't use it *unless* the pt. has *AFib* and CHF.

75. Cc: Sudden, acute CHF in a previously healthy person? → Coxsackie B virus infection

76. Cor Pulmonale ("heart disease due to lungs") refers to impaired RV function due to pulmonary hypertension that occurs as a result of underlying pulmonary disease (e.g., COPD, pulmonary vasculature disease, obstructive sleep apnea).

77. High output cardiac failure will see increased diastolic pressure in LV. Due to:
    a. Arteriovenous fistula – increased preload, increased cardiac output
    b. Hyperthyroidism
    c. Paget disease
    d. Anemia
    e. Thiamine deficiency (Beriberi)

78. Abnormal RBC's
    a. Burr cells (echinocytes) – liver disease, ESRD
    b. Howell-Jolly bodies – Sickle cell pts post splenectomy, amyloidosis, MDS
    c. Spur cells (acanthocytes) – liver disease
    d. Target cells – thalassemia's, chronic liver disease
    e. Schistocytes (fragmented rbc's) – HUS, TTP, DIC, *Scleroderma renal crisis*

79. How do you know Electroconvulsive therapy (ECT) worked? → Will see increased delta waves. Only contraindication is increased intracranial pressure.

80. tPA can be used if <3 hours for a stroke or <12 hours for STEMI

81. Post-MI syncope due to
    a. "Immediate" (10 mins or less) or phase 1a ventricular arrhythmias → reentrant ventricular arrhythmias (ex: VFib)
    b. "Delayed" (10+ mins) or phase 1b arrhythmias → abnormal automaticity

82. Ejection Fraction is a measure of contractility

83. Pneumococcal polysaccharide vaccine (PPSV23)
    a. No memory cells formed (T cell independent B cell response)
    b. Less effective in young, elderly, and immunocompromised
    c. Target demographic is adults <65 yo

84. Pneumococcal conjugate (polysaccharide and protein) vaccine (PCV13)
    a. Memory cells formed (T cell dependent B cell response)
    b. Given to all infants and young children
    c. Given to elderly (65+) and immunocompromised
    d. Bottom line: Babies and kids only get the PCV13, Normal adults only get the PPSV23, Elderly and immunocompromised can get both.

85. Can do D&C for a stillbirth only up to 24 weeks

86. In women with prior history of c-section, use transcervical foley bulb for cervical ripening, NOT misoprostol (increased risk for uterine rupture).

87. Pregnant woman with twins should NOT exercise at all!

88. Alveolar-arterial (A-a) gradient. Normal is 5-15 mm Hg

89. Increased A-a gradient (lots of O2 in alveoli, but can't get into arteries)
    a. Pulmonary embolism
    b. Pulmonary edema (or ARDS)
    c. R → L Shunt
    d. Increased FiO2

90. Normal A-a gradient
    a. High altitude (Decreased FiO2)
    b. Hypoventilation conditions (COPD, OSA, CNS depression, Myasthenia Gravis)

91. Mononucleosis (which is viral) *looks like* Strep throat (which is bacterial)!

92. Gestational Trophoblastic Disease = Elevated Beta-HCG causing ovaries to enlarge
    a. Molar pregnancy (hydatidiform mole) is benign, but can transform into Choriocarcinoma (malignant).
    b. Seen in young women

93. Beta-HCG levels
    a. Higher than normal pregnancy in molar pregnancy
    b. Lower than normal pregnancy in ectopic pregnancy

94. First trimester ultrasound is most accurate way to measure gestational age

95. Normal menstruation should resume 10 weeks after delivery

96. Physiologic leukorrhea = normal vaginal discharge, can have squamous cells and PMN's
    a. White or yellow
    b. No foul smell
    c. Occurs in the absence of other symptoms or findings on vaginal exam

97. Normal vaginal pH is 4.5
    a. pH 5.0 → bacterial vaginosis, trichomoniasis
    b. pH 4.5 → candida infection (can't tell infection by pH alone)

98. Pneumonia by gram stain
    a. Gram + cocci in clusters → Staph aureus
    b. Gram +cocci in pairs ("lancet-shaped diplococci") → Strep pneumoniae
    c. Gram – rods (often in older adults) → E. coli
    d. Gram – rods in neonate → E. coli
    e. Gam + cocci in neonate → Group B Strep (GBS)

99. Ovarian cancer = Adnexal mass + Nonspecific GI symptoms (early satiety, constipation/diarrhea, anorexia, bloating/increased abdominal girth).

100. Short cervix is a cervix <2.5 cm in length

101. Test for BRCA or HER2/Neu if a 1st degree relative had breast cancer *before age 50* or ovarian cancer *at any age*.
    a. BRCA – Rx: Tamoxifen reduces risk for breast cancer, OCP reduces risk for ovarian cancer
    b. HER2/Neu – Rx: Trastuzumab. Rare SE: CHF

102. CT Scan, Xray, and IV pyelogram are contraindicated in pregnancy due to fetal exposure to radiation. *Ultrasound and MRI are allowed.*

103. Aromatase (in ovaries and fat tissue) converts androgens into estrogen

104. Urinary retention post-partum = bladder atony

105. At the end of the 2nd trimester (24-28 weeks), the woman should get screened for gestational diabetes.

106. Pseudocyesis (conversion disorder) = woman badly wants to get pregnant. Has symptoms of pregnancy even though she is *not* pregnant!

107. Pulmonary Edema symptoms = orthopnea, cough, rales/crackles

108. SLE can mimic pre-eclampsia
    a. Protein loss in SLE much higher (approximately 8g/24 hr)
    b. Malar rash
    c. +ANA
    d. RBC casts in urine
    e. Hypertension
    f. Edema

109. 2 cm from the cervix is the cut off for placenta previa

110. Fever = 100.4 degrees Fahrenheit

111. Hyperechoic mass on breast = benign

112. Menarche (1st period) after age 13 = decreased breast cancer risk due to decrease in lifetime estrogen exposure.

113. Claw Hand (Klumpke's)
    a. Goes with Horner's syndrome (miosis, ptosis)
    b. Damage to C8 and T1 (ulnar nerve)

    c. * Absent grasp reflex
    d. Intact moro and biceps reflex

114. Erb-Duchenne Palsy
    a. Damage to C5 & C6 (axillary nerve)
    b. Intact grasp reflex
    c. Decreased moro and biceps reflex

115. Hemolytic Uremic Syndrome (HUS)
    a. In children
    b. H/o GI infection
    c. Hematuria, schistocytes
    d. Rx: Self-limited or plasmapheresis. *Do not give antibiotics!*

116. Idiopathic Thrombocytopenic Purpura (ITP)
    a. In women (chronic illness)
    b. H/o viral illness, often URI
    c. Associated with lymphoma, CLL, HIV, connective tissue disorders
    d. Megakaryocytes
    e. Petechiae everywhere
    f. Rx: Steroids, IV Immunoglobulin, Splenectomy (even though spleen is not enlarged)
    g. Newer Rx: Romiplostim, Eltrombopag = thrombopoietin receptor agonists to stimulate platelet production

117. Thrombotic Thrombocytopenic Purpura (TTP)
    a. Due to a deficiency in ADAMTS-13
    b. "FAT RN" = Fever, Anemia *(MAHA)*, Thrombocytopenia, Renal pathology, Neuro symptoms (headache, seizure, ams). All symptoms do not need to be present at the same time.
    c. Microangiopathic Hemolytic Anemia + low platelets is TTP until proven otherwise.
    d. Rx: Plasmapheresis

118. CHF has a *productive* cough

119. Squamous cell carcinoma of lungs produces PTHrp (but PTH levels will be normal) → hypercalcemia (inhibits ADH, so frequent urination seen). "stones, bones, groans, thrones, and psychiatric overtones"

120. Adenocarcinoma of lung's paraneoplastic syndrome?
    a. Hypertrophic osteoarthropathy (Bamberger-Marie syndrome) = clubbing of fingers + painful ankles and wrists + increased bone deposition on long bones

121. Amniotic fluid embolism (occurs just after delivery)

a. =hypoxemic respiratory failure + severe hypotension + cardiogenic shock + DIC (purpura) + seizures.
   b. Risk factors: advanced maternal age, high gravida
   c. Rx: intubation + mechanical ventilation

122. Large cell carcinoma of the lungs = rare, peripheral lesion. Associated with gynecomastia, galactorrhea.

123. Normal pleural fluid pH = 7.60
   a. Transudate pH = 7.40-7.55 (basic)
   b. Exudate pH = 7.30-7.45 (acidic)
   c. Empyema, tumor, pleural fibrosis pH < 7.30

124. Interstitial lung disease and COPD can cause multifocal atrial tachycardia. Rx for this tachycardia: verapamil or metoprolol

125. Severe renal insufficiency has GFR < 30
   a. Low molecular weight heparin (enoxaparin) or Factor Xa inhibitor (rivaroxaban, fondaparinux) can't be used if the pt. has severe renal insufficiency.
   b. Must use unfractionated heparin instead in this situation

126. Pleural effusion seen on chest xray, next step?
   a. Thoracentesis to determine transudate vs. exudate

127. Remember that elevated wbc count can also be due to *stress*

128. Pneumonia can cause pleural effusion

129. Tuberous Sclerosis → Infantile spasms or seizures (West Syndrome). Rx: ACTH or Vigabatrin

130. Metformin is renal excretion so it should not be used while undergoing CT with contrast
   a. Stop metformin at time of procedure
   b. Withhold metformin for 48 hours subsequent to procedure
   c. Reinstate metformin only after renal fraction has been re-evaluated and found to be normal.

131. Heparin only for *active* thrombus or embolism
   a. Warfarin to ppx against stroke if AFib present
   b. Aspirin to ppx against stroke (general prevention)

132. Amyotrophic Lateral Sclerosis aka Lou Gehrig's Disease (ALS)
   a. UMN signs – spasticity, bulbar symptoms (dysphagia), hyperreflexia, clonus, +Babinski
   b. LMN signs – Fasciculations

133. Deep Tendon Reflexes (DTR's) *are* present even in brain death, since spinal cord is still functioning.

134. Hypertensive emergency = BP > 180/120. Signs: n/v, headache, confusion. Rx: Sodium nitroprusside injection (1st line), Labetalol (2nd line)

135. Greenish breast discharge + nipple retraction + pain = Mammary duct ectasia

136. Phenylephrine causes vasoconstriction, but with bradycardia

137. Ddx: Desquamation of hands and feet in children
    a. Scarlet Fever
    b. Kawasaki Disease
    c. Toxic Shock Syndrome
    d. Stevens-Johnson Syndrome
    e. Acrodynia (from mercury toxicity)

138. Anti-cholinergic symptoms (as seen in benztropine, trihexyphenidyl use)
    a. Flushing, anhidrosis, dry mouth, hyperthermia, mydriasis, delirium/confusion, urinary retention, constipation, headache, dizziness, tachycardia.
    b. Note: Trihexyphenidyl has the se of acute glaucoma

139. Intracerebral hemorrhagic strokes occur at basal ganglia (putamen) and internal capsule (both anterior and posterior limbs involved)

140. Diabetes can damage the eyes at CN III (ptosis and down and out gaze) via *nerve ischemia*. However, accommodation and light reflex are unaffected.

141. Alpha-1 antitrypsin deficiency → liver biopsy shows hepatocytes that are PAS+ and Diastase resistant.

142. Wilson's Disease = Parkinsonism (resting tremor, muscular rigidity, clumsy gait) + excess copper. Rx: Penicillamine

143. +Babinski sign (plantar extension = hyperreflexia = toes spread up and out) = corticospinal lesion = UMN lesion

144. +Romberg sign = proprioception lesion = dorsal column lesion

145. Pediatric Glycogen Storage Disorders are frequently tested and easily confused. The four disorders below should be thoroughly memorized.

146. Type I (Von Gierke) – deficiency in Glucose 6-Phosphatase
    a. Increased glycogen in liver, severe fasting, hypoglycemia
    b. Severe hepatosplenomegaly, enlarged kidneys
    c. Lactic acidosis, hyperlipidemia, hyperuricemia (gout)

d. Doll-like face with wasting extremities
   e. Rx: Cornstarch

147. Type II (Pompe) – deficiency in Acid Maltase (Lysosomal alpha-1, 4-glucosidase)
   a. Diaphragm weakness → Respiratory failure
   b. Hypotonia ("floppy baby syndrome"), dysphagia, macroglossia, hepatomegaly
   c. Cardiomegaly ("Pompe trashes the pump")
   d. Rx: Myozyme (algucosidase alpha)

148. Type III (Cori) – deficiency in Debranching Enzyme/Glucosidase (Amylo-Alpha-1, 6-glucosidase)
   a. Hepatomegaly, hypoglycemia, hyperlipidemia, stunted growth
   b. NORMAL kidneys, normal levels of lactic acid and uric acid
   c. Rx: High protein diet to facilitate gluconeogenesis + Vitamin D to prevent osteoporosis.

149. Type V (McArdle) – deficiency in Glycogen Phosphorylase
   a. Painful muscle cramps, myoglobinuria with strenuous exercise
   b. NORMAL lactic acid
   c. Rx: Oral sucrose before exercise

150. XXX Syndrome → cc: female child in 80th percentile for height and 20th percentile for head circumference.

151. Phenylketonuria (PKU)
   a. The enzyme (phenylalanine hydroxylase) that converts Phenylalanine to Tyrosine is deficient. Therefore, Phenylalanine builds up in the blood.
   b. Mental retardation, stunted growth, seizures, fair skin, eczema, musty body odor
   c. Rx: Decrease phenylalanine and increase tyrosine in the diet, Tetrahydrobiopterin supplementation

152. Papilledema – caused by increased intracranial pressure → compresses optic nerve sheath resulting in swelling of the optic nerve head. Can cause momentary vision loss that varies according to changes in head positioning.

153. Xanthochromia = presence of bilirubin in the CSF = CSF from a lumbar puncture turning *yellow* = only positive marker the pt. is suffering an acute subarachnoid hemorrhage (SAH).

154. Focal Neurological Deficits (FND)
   a. Hemiplegia = Hemiparesis = paralysis (both words mean exactly the same)
   b. Hemisensory deficits
   c. Slurred speech
   d. Aphasia

155. A MMSE score < 24 suggests dementia

156. Sick euthyroid syndrome → normal TSH, abnormal T4/T3

157. Subclinical hypothyroidism → Elevated TSH, normal T4/T3

158. Thyrotropin-releasing Hormone (TRH) suppresses Growth Hormone (GH) levels in normal individuals, but causes a paradoxical increase in GH levels in 50-60% of pts with acromegaly.

159. Cc: Alcoholic with cirrhosis, elevated BUN, hypoalbuminemia, hyponatremia?
    a. Hepatic encephalopathy

160. Long-term use of glucocorticoids (steroids) can lead to
    a. Central adrenal insufficiency→ shuts down CRH and ACTH
    b. Osteoporosis
    c. Proximal muscle weakness

161. Hypocalcemia can be caused by
    a. Respiratory alkalosis – Ionized Ca binds to albumin since H ions kicked off albumin. Remember that albumin in blood lowers Ca levels.
    b. Blood transfusions with *citrate* → binds to ionized Ca, esp. if hepatic dysfunction present (liver clears citrate).
    c. Ca chelation -via lactate, foscarnet, EDTA

162. Lymphomas cause increased 1,25-OH vitamin D production, which in turn causes increased gut Ca absorption leading to hypercalcemia.

163. Bone pain + increased Alk Phos?
    a. Osteomalacia (Increased PTH (secondary hyperparathyroidism), Decreased Ca and Phosphorous)
    b. Paget's disease of the bone (Normal levels of PTH, Ca, and Phosphorous)

164. Delayed hemolytic reaction
    a. Caused by antibodies to Kidd or RhD antigens
    b. Occurs 2-10 days post transfusion
    c. Causes slight fever, less-severe hemolysis, mild increase in unconjugated bilirubin
    d. Rx: None needed; determine what antibody caused it to prevent future reactions

165. Blood deficiency and what to give in transfusion

Blood deficiency	What to give in transfusion
Severe anemia due to autoimmune hemolytic anemia.	pRBC's
Hemophilia	Factor 8 for A, Factor 9 for B
DIC	FFP, platelets
Shock due to trauma or postpartum hemorrhage.	pRBC's, IV fluids

To maintain bp during large volume paracentesis	Albumin
Hemorrhage due to warfarin overdose	FFP + Vitamin K
Need for vWF rich blood product	Cryoprecipitate
Thrombocytopenia	Platelets

166. Mannitol reduces intracranial pressure, but the se is increased sodium (hypernatremia)

167. Hypothyroidism – increased systemic vascular resistance (SVR) leading to HTN

168. Hyperthyroidism – decreased SVR, but bp rises due to increased inotropy (increased contractility) and chronotropy (increased heart rate).

169. "Facial plethora" = Cushing Syndrome

170. ACE-I best to slow diabetic nephropathy and decrease microalbuminuria

171. FeNA < 1 is Pre-Renal Failure.
    a. FeNa > 2 is Intrinsic renal failure

172. Flail Chest = paradoxical breathing due to rib fracture
    a. Rx: O2 + BiPAP or endotracheal intubation w/ mechanical ventilation + Analgesia (limited breathing from pain can lead to hypoxia).

173. Annual diabetes screening
    a. Anyone ≥ 45 years old
    b. BP ≥ 135/80
    c. Risk factors: smoking, dyslipidemia (low HDL, high LDL), HTN, PCOS

174. Cc: Post-anesthesia induction → severe HTN + pallor due to vasoconstriction from catecholamines?
    a. Pheochromocytoma

175. SAAG Score = Serum Albumin – Ascites Fluid Albumin
    a. SAAG > 1.1 means ascites is from a portal HTN related cause (cirrhosis, right-sided CHF, Budd-Chiari syndrome). Increased capillary hydrostatic pressure.
    b. SAAG < 1.1 means ascites is from cancer, TB, pancreatitis, or nephrotic syndrome. Increased capillary permeability.

176. Acute Abdomen → Causes of Bowel Obstruction "HANG IV"
    a. Hernias, Adhesions, Neoplasms, Gallstone Ileus, Intussusception, Volvulus

177. Most common adverse reactions of various immunosuppressants

Immunosuppressant	Adverse Reaction
Muromonab-CD3	Leukopenia
Rapamycin	Thrombocytopenia, Hyperlipidemia

Mycophenolate	Leukopenia, **Lymphoma**, Teratogenic
Hydroxychloroquine	Visual disturbances
Tacrolimus	Nephrotoxicity

178. Pts who have life-threatening *egg allergies* should not receive the MMR vaccine

179. Fracture associations

Fracture	Association
Anterior Shoulder dislocation	Axillary nerve injury (C5, C6)
Humerus fracture	Radial nerve injury
Tibia fracture	Compartment Syndrome

180. VSD = holosystolic murmur at left lower sternal border (cc: Edwards Syndrome)
    a. ASD = Systolic ejection murmur (fixed split S2) at left upper sternal border
    b. PDA = Harsh, holosystolic murmur at left sub-clavicular region

181. Thymus = "sail sign" on child <3 year old's xray

182. Truncus arteriosus is strongly linked to Di George Syndrome ("CATCH 22"). **C**ardiac abnormality (TOF), **A**bnormal facies, **T**hymic aplasia (leads to T cell deficiency), **C**left palate, **H**ypocalcemia. **22q11** deletion. The thymus and parathyroids both don't develop in Di George Syndrome!

183. PANDAS = Pediatric Autoimmune Neuropsychiatric Disorders Associated with Streptococcal infections.
    a. Cc: OCD that occurs post strep infection in a child
    b. Rx: SSRI for OCD, Risperidone if tics present

184. Earliest sign of compartment syndrome?
    a. Pain with passive motion

185. Depression + Neuropathic Pain? → Rx: Duloxetine

186. Mullerian ducts = Fallopian tubes, uterus, upper 1/3 of vagina. Ovaries <u>not</u> included.
    a. Rx for Mullerian agenesis? Elevate the vagina

187. Lyme disease rx
    a. In children <8 years old → Amoxicillin
    b. In adults → Doxycycline
    c. For rx of CNS Lyme disease + Heart block → IV Ceftriaxone

188. CD 19+ = B Cells. Low in SCID, Absent in Bruton's X-linked agammaglobulinemia

189. CD 3+ = T Cells. Absent in SCID, Normal in Bruton's X-linked agammaglobulinemia

190. Cc: Boy falls while brushing teeth, develops hemiparesis → Carotid artery dissection

191. Teriparatide (anabolic bone growing agent) is a pulsatile (activates osteoblasts > osteoclasts) PTH analog that can be used to treat osteoporosis.

192. Cc: Knee x-ray reveals calcification of menisci → Pseudogout (deposits Ca into articular joints)

193. Osteopetrosis
    a. Cc: Narrowing of the bone marrow cavity results in low H&H
    b. Osteoclast dysfunction
    c. Carbonic anhydrase defect. Increased ALP
    d. Rx: bone marrow transplant

194. Pyuria ≥ 5 wbc/hpf
    a. Bacteriuria = 50,000 cfu/ml from a catheterized specimen

195. Systolic Ejection Murmurs
    a. Aortic Stenosis
    b. Atrial Septal Defect (ASD)
    c. Hypertrophic Obstructive Cardiac Myopathy (HOCM)
    d. Tetralogy of Fallot (TOF)
    e. Truncus Arteriosus

196. Tricuspid Regurgitation, Mitral Regurgitation, and VSD all have a holosystolic murmur

197. Atopic dermatitis is another name for eczema. Due to improper synthesis of stratum corneum.

198. Cancers that metastasize to the bones: "BLT with a Kosher Pickle"
    a. Breast (either blastic or lytic), Lung (lytic), Thyroid, Kidney, Prostate (blastic)

199. Anemia of Chronic Disease: Increased IL-6 → Increased Hepcidin from Liver → Decreased Ferroportin (iron carrier protein) → Decreased iron in circulation.

200. Systemic Lupus Erythematosus (SLE)
    a. Painless oral ulcers
    b. +ANA
    c. Decreased C3 and C4
    d. Drug induced Lupus has anti-histone antibodies. For the drugs think "SHIPP"
        i. Sulfonamides, Hydralazine, Isoniazid, Phenytoin, Procainamide

201. Organophosphates inhibit ACH-esterase → Increased ACH
    a. Rx: Atropine (inhibits ACH receptor) + 2-PAM (regenerates ACH-esterase)
        i. Rx for *atropine* overdose is Physostigmine (ACH-esterase inhibitor)

202. Aspirin increases bleeding time because it decreases platelet function, *but* platelet count is normal. PT and PTT are also normal.

203. Bernard-Soulier = deficiency in GpIb (receptor for vW Factor). Has decreased platelet count, increased bleeding time.
    a. Rx: FFP

204. Glanzmann's Thrombasthenia = GpIIb/IIIa defect (receptor on platelets). Normal platelet count, increased bleeding time.
    a. Rx: Recombinant factor VIIa

205. "Sacroiliitis" or "Sacral-Iliitis" on the USMLE means Ankylosing Spondylitis (can occur in other conditions, but use this association for test purposes).
    a. Cc: pain worse in the AM and following inactivity

206. The knee-chest position in TOF increases *systemic* vascular resistance

207. Rare se of Rotavirus vaccine?
    a. Intussusception

208. In neonate<28 days, to rx bacterial meningitis instead of ceftriaxone use cefotaxime. Ceftriaxone displaces bilirubin from albumin and increases risk for kernicterus.

209. Prematurity and maternal diabetes are the biggest risk factors for respiratory distress syndrome (RDS) of the newborn.
    a. Insulin blocks the maturation of sphingomyelin
    b. Maternal diabetes also increases the risk for Transposition of the Great Vessels

210. Treat the *close contacts* of the sick in the following conditions
    a. Pertussis – Rx: azithromycin, clarithromycin, erythromycin
    b. Epiglottitis – Rx: Rifampin

211. If the electrolyte disturbances are not corrected before surgery in pyloric stenosis, then *apnea* can result.

212. Any cyanotic (R → L) congenital heart disease increases the risk for brain abscess. Will see multiple abscesses along distribution of MCA (gray-white matter junction).

213. Hypothermia in a neonate is t< 96.8 degrees Fahrenheit. Think sepsis if you see this.

214. Vasculitis = destruction of blood vessels by T cells

215. Constitutional B Signs (fever, night sweats, weight loss) seen in what conditions?
    a. Cancer, TB, Lymphoma, Waldenstrom Macroglobulinemia

216. Menses

    a. Estrogen builds up the endometrium
    b. Progesterone breaks down the endometrium

217. Beckwith-Wiedemann Syndrome associated with:
    a. Wilms Tumor – dx: abdominal ultrasound
    b. Hepatoblastoma – dx: AFP level
    c. Omphalocele

218. All infants receive Hepatitis B vaccine <u>at birth</u> as long as baby is at least 4 lbs. All other vaccines start at 2 months.

219. Bedwetting should be done by age 5

220. Normal birth weight is 5.5-10.0 lbs

221. Bilious vs. Non-Bilious vomiting conditions

Bilious vomiting	Non-Bilious vomiting
Duodenal atresia	Pyloric stenosis
Intestinal (Jejunal) atresia	Intussusception
Annular pancreas	
Malrotation (Volvulus)	
Meconium ileus	
Hirschsprung's disease	
Necrotizing enterocolitis	

222. Haptoglobin binds free hemoglobin. Haptoglobin-Hb complexes are removed by the spleen. Haptoglobin levels decrease in hemolytic anemia.

223. The edema in Turner Syndrome is due to dysgenesis/underdevelopment of lymphatic system.

224. Sinusitis = swelling of nasal turbinates, nasal discharge

225. CAH (21-OH deficiency) causes advanced bone and accelerated growth (increased height).

226. Hydrocele will transilluminate light, other testicular masses will not. There is a risk for *inguinal hernia* if it doesn't recede by 12 months of age.

227. Renal Tubular Acidosis (RTA) = Normal anion gap metabolic acidosis
    a. Check urinary anion gap (urine sodium + urine potassium – urine chloride)
    b. If urinary anion gap > +10, then RTA is present

228. Serum osmoles = $(2 \times Na) + Glucose/18 + BUN/2.8$. [Normal is 280]

229. Glomerulonephritis (general term) = dysmorphic rbc's, blood + protein in urine. Further classify into nephritic and nephrotic syndromes.

230. Nephritic Syndrome – <u>hematuria</u>, HTN, oliguria, increased creatinine, increased nitrogen in blood.

231. Nephrotic Syndrome – <u>proteinuria</u>, edema, <u>fatty casts</u>, hyperlipidemia, increased risk of infection, increased risk of thromboembolism.

232. NSAID use can cause SIADH

233. Increased bleeding (ex: GI bleed) → Increased BUN since blood is converted to urea (along with other breakdown products like bilirubin)

234. Metabolic Alkalosis. HCO3 > 28
    a. Urine Chloride > 20 (not volume responsive)
        i. +HTN → Conn's syndrome, Renal Artery Stenosis
        ii. -HTN → Bartter's syndrome, Gitelman's syndrome
    b. Urine Chloride < 20 (volume responsive)
        i. Diuretics
        ii. Emesis (vomiting acid)
        iii. Dehydration
        iv. NG Suction used

235. Low complement (C3) + Renal Disease
    a. PSGN (Post-streptococcal glomerulonephritis)
    b. MPGN (Membranoproliferative glomerulonephritis)
    c. Lupus nephritis
    d. Mixed cryoglobulinemia associated with Hepatitis C

236. Acute transplant rejection → Give IV steroids STAT

237. BPH = smooth, enlarged, firm prostate

238. Prostate Cancer = palpable nodule at the periphery of the prostate

239. Lactic Acidosis (LA)
    a. Transient LA seen after a *seizure* (as an anion gap metabolic acidosis)
    b. Hypotension with poor end organ perfusion may cause LA → Rx: Dopamine

240. Ureterovesical junction = where the ureter meets the bladder
    a. Ureteropelvic junction = where the ureter attaches to the kidney

241. Microhematuria is ≥ 3 rbc/hpf

242. Hepatorenal syndrome

a. No blood, protein, or casts seen in urine
   b. Pts do not respond to IV fluids and withdrawal of diuretics

243. SLE and Kidney Disease
   a. Nephrotic Syndrome (Membranous Glomerulonephritis) – Normal C3 and C4
   b. Nephritic Syndrome (Lupus Nephritis) – Low C3 and C4
      i. Photosensitive skin (sunburn)
      ii. Renal failure
      iii. Rbc's and Protein in urine

244. What is mcc of death in dialysis pts? → Cardiovascular (CHF, MI, etc.)

245. Hyperphosphatemia often present in dialysis pts, give Calcium to correct

246. Lactic Acidosis (seen in states of hypoperfusion)
   a. Sepsis
   b. Shock
   c. Cyanide poisoning
   d. End Stage Liver Disease

247. Another name for normal saline (0.9% NaCl) is "crystalloid" solution. IV colloids (albumin) are used to treat burns or hypoproteinemia.

248. SAAG< 1.1 means increased capillary permeability
   a. Cancer
   b. TB
   c. Pancreatitis
   d. Nephrotic Syndrome

249. Hyponatremia workup
   a. Serum Osmolality > 290 → Yes → Hyperglycemia, Advanced Renal Failure
   b. If No, is Urine Osmolality < 100 → Yes → Primary Polydipsia, Beer Potomania
   c. If No, is Urine Sodium > 25
      i. Yes: SIADH, Adrenal insufficiency (losing Na due to lack of aldosterone), Hypothyroidism.
      ii. No: Volume depletion, CHF, Cirrhosis

250. Acetazolamide treats metabolic alkalosis by inhibiting carbonic anhydrase, leads to decreased reabsorption of HCO3. Se: hypokalemia, metabolic acidosis.

251. Normal post void residual volume (PVR) for men < 50 ml, for women < 150 ml

252. Cirrhosis only has lower extremity edema (ascites); there is no pulmonary edema (JVP not elevated).

253. Ascites with SAAG > 1.1 = Cirrhosis = Portal Hypertension = Increased capillary hydrostatic pressure = nonperitoneal cause of ascites
    a. Right heart failure, constrictive pericarditis, Budd-Chiari syndrome
    b. Portal hypertension leads to thrombocytopenia secondary to splenomegaly, as platelets are sequestered in the liver.

254. SAAG score = Serum albumin – Ascites albumin

255. Esophageal cancer metastasizes early because the esophagus lacks a serosa

256. Stress Ulcers – both types can cause acute gastritis
    a. Curling ulcer – due to burn injury
    b. Cushing ulcer – due to traumatic brain injury

257. Misoprostol can help patients with peptic ulcer disease (PUD) who require NSAID therapy (e.g., for arthritis)

258. Chronic diarrhea in HIV/AIDS pts? → Cryptosporidium and Isospora

259. Carcinoid syndrome can lead to Pellagra. Tryptophan is being converted mainly to Serotonin and not to Niacin (Vitamin B3).

260. Direct hernias lie medial and indirect lie lateral to the inferior epigastric vessels

261. Abnormal LFT's:
    a. Hepatocellular injury: Increased AST and ALT
    b. Cholestasis: Increased Alkaline Phosphatase (ALP) and Bilirubin

262. Cc: Woman who reports chronic biliary colic. Labs show elevated AST, ALT, Lipids?
    a. Gallstone pancreatitis

263. Nonalcoholic Steatohepatitis (NASH) associated with metabolic syndrome and insulin resistance. Rx: Vitamin E, Pioglitazone

264. Sorafenib to rx advanced metastatic hepatocellular carcinoma, renal cell carcinoma, and thyroid cancer. MOA: tyrosine kinase (C-RAF) inhibitor that induces autophagy.

265. Chronic Hepatitis C infection is associated with:
    a. Intermittent elevation of AST, ALT
    b. Porphyria Cutanea Tarda (PCT) = fragile skin, hyperpigmentation, photosensitivity, hypertrichosis, vesicles and erosions on dorsum of hand.
    c. Essential Mixed Cryoglobulinemia = palpable purpura, arthralgias, membranoproliferative glomerulonephritis, low C3.

266. Rebound tenderness and guarding is seen in appendicitis and peritonitis

267. Hepatic encephalopathy (asterixis, confusion) is present in acute liver failure, but not in acute hepatitis.

268. Phenobarbital can reduce serum bilirubin in Crigler-Najar Type 2 (but not in Type 1) by inducing hepatic enzymes.

269. Acute pancreatitis can cause pleural effusion

270. Cc: Man comes in tired, labs show Hb <7. What to do? → PRBC transfusion

271. Pregnancy
    a. Estrogen causes increased cholesterol secretion
    b. Progesterone causes decreased bile acid secretion and slows gallbladder emptying
    c. The effect of both hormones leads to cholesterol gallstones

272. Hepatitis A
    a. Cc: Aversion to smoking
    b. Give close contacts IVIG

273. Drug induced liver injury – signs are rash, arthralgia, fever, leukocytosis, eosinophilia. The listed drugs cause the following conditions:
    a. Cholestasis – chlorpromazine, nitrofurantoin, erythromycin, anabolic steroids
    b. Fatty liver – tetracycline, valproate, anti-retrovirals
    c. Hepatitis – halothane, phenytoin, INH, alpha-methyldopa
    d. Toxic/Fulminant liver failure – carbon tetrachloride, acetaminophen
    e. Granulomatous – allopurinol and phenylbutazone

274. Succussion/gastric splash = sloshing sound heard through the stethoscope during sudden movement of the pt. on abdominal auscultation. It reflects the presence of gas and fluid in an obstructed organ, as in *gastric outlet obstruction* (pyloric stenosis, PUD, gastric cancer are causes).

275. Achalasia takes 5 years to develop until symptoms are noticeable
    a. Pseudoachalasia due to esophageal cancer takes <6 months until symptoms are felt.
        i. "Widened mediastinum" appearance due to tumor metastasis to mediastinal lymph nodes seen on xray.

276. Cor Pulmonale has a prominent "a" wave

277. Lupus = big joints, asymmetric, non-erosive
    a. RA = small joints, symmetric (bilateral), erosive

278. Cryoglobulins are *proteins* (mainly immunoglobulins) that become insoluble at cold temperature.
    a. Cold agglutinins are *IgM* directed against RBC's

279. Hepatitis B + Vasculitis = Polyarteritis Nodosa (PAN)
    a. Hepatitis C + Palpable Purpura + Cryoglobulins = Cryoglobulinemia

280. Polymyalgia Rheumatica
    a. Aching and stiffness in the shoulders, neck, and hips
    b. Elevated ESR associated with anemia
    c. Fever, malaise, weight loss
    d. Rx: Low dose prednisone (10-20 mg/day)

281. C spine subluxation can lead to spinal cord compression in RA
    a. Subluxation + spinal cord compression = hyperreflexia or upgoing-toes on Babinski.

282. Tenosynovitis of the palms ("trigger finger") = RA

283. DMARD's = methotrexate, hydroxychloroquine, sulfasalazine, leflunomide, azathioprine

284. If you suspect Raynaud's phenomenon, order ANA first. Should be negative. However, if positive ANA, then test for CREST's other markers (anti-topoisomerase-1 for systemic sclerosis).

285. Hemochromatosis can cause osteoarthritis. Associated with DM, hypothyroidism, and pseudogout.

286. Low-dose prednisone is the rx for polymyalgia rheumatica

287. Anti-smooth muscle antibodies are seen in what conditions?
    a. Autoimmune hepatitis – can lead to liver failure, acute cirrhosis, Type 1 DM

288. Hyperparathyroidism → Elevated Calcium → Pseudogout (chondrocalcinosis)

289. Arthritis + Nephrotic Syndrome = SLE

290. These is brief (15 minutes) morning stiffness in the arthritis of SLE

291. Valgus stress test worsens pain of Medial Collateral Ligament (MCL) tear

292. Whipple's disease: PAS+ macrophages, non-acid fast gram+ bacilli
    a. HIV+ MAC: PAS+ macrophages, acid fast bacilli

293. Osteoarthritis and Psoriatic arthritis both affect the distal interphalangeal joints (DIP)

294. Cyclophosphamide produces the toxic metabolite acrolein, which causes hemorrhagic cystitis and bladder cancer.

a. Rx: MESNA, fluids

295. Normal Alkaline Phosphatase (ALP): Males 30-100, Females 45-115

296. Spondyloarthropathies = enthesitis = inflammation at sites of *ligamentous* insertion

297. Septic arthritis is more likely if the joint already has OA, RA, Gout or is a prosthetic joint

298. Biologics (infliximab, etanercept, adalimumab, etc.) are anti-cytokine agents that work by interfering with the proinflammatory cytokine TNF-alpha.

299. Primary hyperparathyroidism
    a. Elevated: calcium, ALP, urinary hydroxyproline
    b. Decreased: phosphate

300. Polycythemia Vera leads to gout

301. Carpal Tunnel Syndrome
    a. Pain can radiate to the forearm
    b. Diabetes and obesity are risk factors
    c. Decreased sensation in 1st 3.5 digits
    d. Weakness of thumb opposition
    e. Dx: Nerve conduction studies
    f. Rx: Splint, corticosteroid injection, surgery

302. SE of TNF-alpha inhibitors?
    a. Demyelination, malignancy, infection, CHF

303. Complications of giant cell arteritis?
    a. Aortic aneurysm, blindness

304. Polymyalgia Rheumatica rx?
    a. Low dose oral prednisone

305. Cc: "Popping" sound at knee + hemarthrosis → ACL injury

306. If hypernatremia with hypotension → Rx: 0.9% NS
    a. If hypernatremia with normal bp → Rx: D5W in 0.45% NS

307. Patients with HIV/AIDS and Parkinson's Disease can develop severe *seborrheic dermatitis* (due to Malassezia furfur). Looks like red, scaly patches around ears, eyes, and nasolabial fold.

308. Eczema herpeticum is a medical emergency (HSV can spread to the brain)!
    a. Rx: IV acyclovir

309. Rash involving the extensor surfaces (elbows, knees) → Psoriasis
    a. Rash involving the flexor surfaces (parts of the skin that touch when a joint bends) → Atopic dermatitis (Eczema)

310. Crepitus (gas in tissue) on physical exam + severe pain = Necrotizing Fasciitis

311. A large inflammatory boggy mass caused by tinea capitis is called a Kerion

312. Gas gangrene (C. perfringens) is associated with *dirty wounds* (contaminated with dirt, bowel/fecal matter, black tar heroin injection).
    a. Rx: Debridement +Hyperbaric O2 + Abx

313. Arsenic exposure is a rare cause of multiple squamous cell carcinomas (SCC) in a palmoplantar distribution.

314. Lentigo - benign hyperplasia of melanocytes; linear in spread. Proliferate in basal layer
    a. Freckles (ephelis) – normal # of melanocytes, increased amount of melanin

315. Discoid lupus – Erythematous, scaling plaques affecting the face, ears, scalp

316. Acanthosis Nigricans is associated with DM and PCOS. Risk of gastric cancer. Skin tags.

317. Sudden-onset, severe psoriasis is associated with HIV

318. Severe seborrheic dermatitis is associated with HIV and Parkinson's Disease

319. Immunosuppression increases the risk for SCC

320. Staphylococcal scalded skin syndrome (SSSS) is seen in children post s. aureus infection. Bullae, +Nikolsky sign, facial edema, perioral crusting, and dehydration are common.

321. Cellulitis spreads slowly (3-4 days)

322. Doxycycline (a tetracycline) can cause a phototoxic drug rxn. Avoid the sun!

323. Tinea Corporis (ringworm) = pruritic rash with a scaly erythematous border and central clearing. Has nothing to do with parasitic worms; it is a fungus! Rx: Terbinafine.

324. Sickle Cell Trait sickles rbc's only under extreme conditions and it will be in the *renal vein*. Thus, increased risk for renal vein thrombosis.

325. Direct Coombs test – detects antibodies *bound* to rbc's

326. Indirect Coombs test – detects antibodies against rbc's that are present *unbound* in serum

327. AML, M3 subtype aka acute promyelocytic leukemia – Auer Rods. Rx: ATRA (Vit. A)

328. AML, M4 and M5 subtypes – Esterase. Gum infiltration (M5), CNS symptoms. Rx: Idarubicin + Ara-C

329. "Myelogenous" = Neutrophils

330. Protein Gap = Serum Protein – Serum Albumin
    a. Normal value is 3
    b. If protein gap > 3 and >10% blasts, then Multiple Myeloma. If not, then MGUS

331. Factor Xa Inhibitors = ApiXaban, RivaroXaban. AdeXanet alfa is the reversal agent

332. LMWH (Enoxaparin) mainly inhibits Factor Xa. Protamine is a weak reversal agent

333. Direct Thrombin Inhibitors = Dabigatran, Argabatran, Bivalirudin. Idarucizumab can reverse Dabigatran.

334. Rituximab is anti-CD20 → Inhibits B Cells → therefore, can't make antibodies

335. Phenytoin can cause Folate malabsorption

336. Haptoglobin binds Hb and transports it to the liver in hemolysis. Thus, it is decreased in hemolysis. Much more decreased in intravascular hemolysis; almost normal in extravascular hemolysis.

337. Citrate in blood transfusions can bind to calcium causing *hypocalcemia* (prolonged QT interval, numbness, perioral tingling)

338. Leukemoid reaction = elevated wbc count as a response to stress or infection. Elevated LAP. Dx: Malignancy has decreased LAP.

339. Lactate dehydrogenase (LDH) is a marker of hemolysis. It is also elevated post MI → peaks at 3-4 days and remains elevated up to 10 days.

340. Stored rbc's gradually lose intracellular potassium to the surrounding solution. This has the potential to cause hyperkalemia. Also, citrate in PRBC can bind to serum calcium and magnesium, causing hypocalcemia and hypomagnesemia.

341. Heparin activates antithrombin III, which in turn inactivates IIa, IXa, Xa ("2, 9, 10")

342. Henoch-Schonlein Purpura is a rare case of purpura without thrombocytopenia

343. Chronic hemolysis (as in sickle cell anemia, hereditary spherocytosis) can consume Folate, leading to Megaloblastic anemia.

344. AngelMan's → **M**om's gene is missing → 2 copies from Dad present

a. **Prader Willi** → **Paternal** gene is missing → 2 copies from Mom present

345. Prostate cancer causes osteoblastic lesions. Dx: detect on bone scan

346. Phenytoin and Phenobarbital impair Folic acid absorption
   a. TMP SMX and Methotrexate cause Folic acid deficiency. Rx: Leucovorin

347. Hemolysis depletes Folic Acid the most
   a. New RBC production post EPO requires iron the most

348. Aplastic anemia = pancytopenia. BM biopsy shows a hypoplastic, fat-filled marrow

349. Pernicious anemia → Gastritis → Gastric Cancer

350. Metamyelocyte is more mature than myelocyte. Metamyelocyte becomes a Band

351. Androgen abuse can cause polycythemia (elevated hematocrit). Also elevated LDL, decreased HDL, and hepatotoxicity.

352. Splenectomy
   a. Vaccines for Strep pneumo, Hib, and Meningitis before the operation
   b. Daily oral Penicillin ppx for 3-5 years post operation

353. Diabetic nephropathy is associated with albuminuria

354. Infectious mononucleosis (EBV)
   a. Fatigue, generalized maculopapular rash, posterior cervical lymphadenopathy, splenomegaly, *palatal petechiae*
   b. Leukocytosis with elevated lymphocytes
   c. Heterophile antibodies may be negative early in the disease!

355. HIV can cause thrombocytopenia

356. Splenic sequestration of platelets occurs in cirrhosis, portal HTN, and sickle cell anemia

357. Pernicious anemia is associated with autoimmune diseases (vitiligo, Hashimoto's, etc.)

358. Homocysteine is converted to Methionine. Folic acid and Vitamin B12 are required for this reaction.

359. If Warfarin is not working in treating acute DVT, switch to RivarXaban (Xa inhibitor)

360. Causes of Polycythemia/Erythrocytosis?
   a. Polycythemia Vera
   b. Obstructive sleep apnea

    c. Osler-Weber-Rendu (Hereditary Hemorrhagic Telangiectasia)
    d. Carbon Monoxide poisoning
    e. Renal cell carcinoma. Produces EPO as a paraneoplastic syndrome

361. Focal Proliferative Glomerulonephritis = Seen in 30% of Lupus Nephritis (SLE causes both protein and blood in urine). SLE causes pancytopenia due to immune mediated destruction of cells.

362. Ineffective hematopoiesis refers to blood cell breakdown in bone marrow before release into the circulation. Seen in thalassemia and myelodysplastic syndrome.

363. Megaloblastic anemia has a low reticulocyte count

364. Hemochromatosis
    a. Hypogonadism, diabetes, cirrhosis, hepatomegaly, dilated cardiomyopathy
    b. Arthralgias due to calcium pyrophosphate crystals → pseudogout

365. Exertional heat stroke →AMS, temperature >105 F, rhabdomyolysis

366. Heat Exhaustion – inadequate. Na and H2O replacement during physical activity. Body can't maintain adequate CO. No CNS dysfunction.

367. Cc: Baby with *PCP Pneumonia* in the first year of life?
    a. Hyper IgM Syndrome

368. Strep viridans is the #1 cause of brain abscess = *solitary*, ring-enhancing lesion

369. Disseminated gonorrhea causes monoarticular septic arthritis, rash, and tenosynovitis

370. Gonorrhea coinfections = HIV, chlamydia, syphilis, Hepatitis B

371. What vaccinations do HIV+ pts require?
    a. Hep B, Strep Pneumo, Varicella, PCV13 (Followed by PPSV23 8 weeks later)

372. CMV Mononucleosis = No pharyngitis, lymphadenopathy, or splenomegaly

373. Cc: In HIV+ patient, prophylaxis against Toxoplasmosis and Pneumocystis jiroveci via TMP-SMX

374. Leprosy = anesthetic skin lesions + *nodular*/painful nerve deformities with decreased sensory and motor activity

375. In an old person post URI, Staph aureus can cause a *cavitary* pneumonia

376. Chloroquine sensitive malaria found only in Mexico, Argentina, Caribbean, Turkey, Iraq

377. Osteomyelitis
    a. Leukocytes (wbc's) may be elevated or <u>normal</u>
    b. Fever is present in only 50% of cases
    c. Back pain → Tenderness to gentle percussion over the spinous process of the involved vertebra is the most reliable sign for spinal osteomyelitis
    d. Elevated ESR is a key lab marker
    e. Dx: MRI. CT guided aspiration and culture to confirm

378. Herpes Zoster rx? → Valacyclovir is preferred. Acyclovir also works

379. Tdap (tetanus, diphtheria, acellular pertussis) vaccine – <u>one</u> lifetime dose for everyone. Follow up with Td vaccine every 10 years. However, pregnant women get Tdap <u>with each pregnancy</u>!

380. Cc: Kaposi's sarcoma (HHV-8): lower extremity edema + oral thrush + drug user

381. Cytomegalovirus (CMV) Retinitis + Esophagitis
    a. In HIV+ pt. with CD4<50
    b. Bloody diarrhea + abdominal pain + fever
    c. Dx: Colonoscopy + biopsy

382. Influenza can turn into Pneumonia 4-5 days later. Due to S. Aureus, Strep Pneumo

383. Cc: Pulmonary symptoms + Meningitis? → Strep Pneumo
    a. Neisseria Meningitis does not cause pulmonary symptoms

384. Serum *beta-D-glucan antigen* can be used to dx blood infection by Candida

385. Alkaline urine has ph > 8.0

386. Epiglottitis caused by Haemophilus influenzae type b (rare now because of vaccination) and <u>Strep. Pyogenes</u>

387. Flu hits hard and <u>suddenly</u> with muscle pain, fever, non-productive cough

388. HACEK organisms cause endocarditis via dental procedures. Enterococci (especially E. Faecalis) cause endocarditis via urinary tract infection (UTI).

389. Glasgow Coma Scale (GCS) → "GCS<8, intubate!"
    a. EYES = 4 letters
    b. VOICE = 5 letters
    c. ARM + LEG = 6 letters (motor response)

390. Tension pneumothorax, sites for needle decompression
    a. 2nd intercostal space in the midclavicular line

b. 5th intercostal space in the midaxillary line

391. Treatment order for hemoptysis:
   a. Bronchoscopy → Pulmonary arteriography → Thoracotomy

392. Alkaline Phosphatase (ALP) elevated in the following conditions:
   a. Cholestasis (extrahepatic bile ducts blocked) → from gallstones, pancreatic cancer, primary sclerosing cholangitis (PSC)
   b. Paget's Disease of the bone
   c. Leukemoid reaction

393. Phenytoin, Carbamazepine, and Rifampin cause Vitamin D deficiency by inducing the Cytochrome P450 system which degrades Vitamin D to inactive metabolites.

394. PEEP mechanical ventilation increases intrathoracic pressure, decreases ventricular preload and venous return to the heart.

395. Atelectasis and Pneumonia on post-op days 1-2 due to shallow breathing and impaired cough reflex. Rx: Incentive spirometer.

396. Cc: "wrist pain and swelling". Rx for non-displaced scaphoid fracture?
   a. Thumb spica cast for 6 weeks

397. Peripheral Arterial Disease (PAD) = narrowing of the arteries other than those that supply the heart or brain.
   a. Cc: The classic symptom is leg pain while walking which resolves with rest = intermittent claudication.
   b. Other signs: cold skin, blue skin, skin ulcers (esp. of leg), poor nail and hair growth.
   c. Main risk factor is smoking
   d. Dx: Ankle-Brachial Index (ABI) ≤ 0.90
      i. ABI ≥ 1.30 suggests calcified and uncompressible vessels → additional vascular studies needed.
   e. Rx: Exercise, smoking cessation, Cilostazol (PDE3 inhibitor, inhibits platelet aggregation), Pentoxifylline (non-selective PDE inhibitor, xanthine derivative)

398. ALT > 150 → Gallstone pancreatitis

399. Necrotizing fasciitis = Deep bacterial infection
   a. Cc: Pain out of proportion to physical exam findings
   b. Signs: Fever, hypotension, erythema, swelling
   c. Diabetes and immunosuppression are major risk factors
   d. Gas production by microbes leads to air in soft tissues → Crepitus
   e. Rx: Surgical debridement + antibiotics

400. Medial Meniscus injury vs. Medial Collateral Ligament (MCL) injury

Medial Meniscus injury	MCL injury
Small joint effusion	From severe valgus stress (lateral injury)
Crepitus, locking, catching with ROM	Ecchymosis and joint line tenderness at medial knee.
Dx: Ege's test	Dx: Valgus stress test

401. Parotid gland surgery can harm Facial (CN 7) Nerve leading to facial droop

402. Strabismus ("crossed eyes") can cause Amblyopia ("lazy eye")
    a. Rx for Amblyopia is to cover the good eye with an eye patch

403. Rx for Flail Chest?
    a. Rx: PEEP + Intubation + Chest tube placement

404. Hypocalcemia can cause QT prolongation

405. Catheterization can cause *retroperitoneal hematoma*
    a. Signs: sudden hemodynamic instability, ipsilateral flank or back pain
    b. Dx: Non-contrast CT of abdomen and pelvis
    c. Rx: Supportive

406. A fall from a height of 10+ feet can cause aortic injury.
    a. Dx: Mediastinal widening, deviation of trachea to right w/NG tube

407. Diabetes mellitus leads to increased risk for necrotizing fasciitis at surgical wound site

408. Fluorescein exam with woods lamp to examine high-velocity eye injuries (from drilling, grinding). Also to see corneal abrasions or Herpes keratitis.

409. Atropine dilates (mydriasis) pupils, therefore avoid using in glaucoma patients

410. Chalazion = granulomatous inflammation of the meibomian gland. Rx: Incision & curettage

411. Open angle glaucoma can lead to optic nerve cupping

412. (Central) Macular degeneration → distortion of straight lines such that they appear wavy

413. Dacryocystitis = infection of the lacrimal sac (medial canthus) by S. aureus or Beta hemolytic strep.

414. Presbycusis = (Bilateral) Sensorineural hearing loss that occurs with aging. Worse hearing high-pitched voices. Mainly in senior adults.

415. Serous otitis media = presence of middle ear effusion without infection

a. Seen in HIV/AIDS pts
  b. Physical Exam: Dull tympanic membrane that is hypomobile
  c. Conductive hearing loss

416. Transverse nasal crease = "allergic salute". Seen in allergic rhinitis

417. Aspirin Exacerbated Respiratory Disease (AERD). Symptoms:
  a. Asthma
  b. Chronic rhinosinusitis with recurrent nasal polyps
  c. Bronchospasm following the ingestion of aspirin or NSAID
  d. Anosmia

418. Malignant otitis externa → Seen in old, diabetic pts
  a. Caused by Pseudomonas infection
  b. Granulation tissue in auditory canal
  c. Pain chewing food due to osteomyelitis of TMJ
  d. CN 7 palsy

419. Cc: Heavy, prolonged, intermenstrual or postmenopausal bleeding = endometrial hyperplasia or cancer

420. Cc: Losing weight in pregnancy, how?
  a. Hyperemesis gravidarum
  b. Dx: ketonuria

421. Blood is absorbed in hemorrhage
  a. Increase in BUN results
  b. Bun/Cr > 20 indicates upper GI bleed

422. Decreased haptoglobin + Increased LDH → Hemolytic Anemia

423. Hospice care = Can be own home, assisted living facility, or dedicated living facility. Requires survival prognosis of ≤ 6 months.

424. In experimental studies, you fix the problem of confounding via stratification

425. NPV and PPV varies with the pretest probability of a disease

426. Advanced Sleep Phase Syndrome = You fall asleep early (around 7 pm). Can't stay awake at night.

427. Delayed Sleep Phase Syndrome = You are a night owl. You can't fall asleep. Wake up tired.

428. "Bath Salts" = Synthetic cathinones

      a. Can't be detected by urine toxicology
      b. Effects (psychosis, severe agitation) *last one week*

429. Pt with a single episode of Major Depressive Disorder (MDD) should continue antidepressants for an additional 4-9 months following symptom resolution.

430. Catatonia rx is benzodiazepine (lorazepam) or ECT

431. Gender dysphoria = persistent (≥ 6 months) incongruence between assigned and felt gender.
      a. Rx: medication to delay puberty. Gender reassignment surgery after 18 years old

432. "Ecstasy"/"E"/"Molly"/MDMA use can cause hyponatremia. "Dance so much you sweat out the salt"

433. Cryoglobulinemia = proteins in the blood that become insoluble at cold temperature. Fingers and toes become gangrenous.
      a. Cc #1: Hepatitis C + Cryoglobulins + Palpable Purpura
          i. Dx: Decreased C4
      b. Cc #2: Waldenstrom Macroglobulinemia
      c. Cc #3: Multiple Myeloma

434. Cold Hemagglutinin aka Cold AIHA = IgM antibodies against rbc's in cold temperature
      a. This is a Coombs+ hemolytic anemia
      b. Cc #1 (kids): EBV, Mycoplasma Pneumonia
      c. Cc #2 (adults): CLL, Waldenstrom Macroglobulinemia

435. Can't be detected by drug screens:
      a. Bath salts (synthetic cathinones) – Makes you go into a rage
      b. Inhalants (toluene) – Makes you euphoric
          i. MOA: CNS depressant
          ii. Dx: Rash seen around mouth or nostrils

436. Glucocorticoids at high dose can induce psychosis, mania, or depression

437. Neuroleptic Malignant Syndrome (NMS) – due to adverse rxn from anti-psychotic drug
      a. Signs: muscle rigidity, <u>fever</u>, autonomic instability, delirium
      b. Labs: Elevated ck and wbc
      c. Rx: Remove the offending drug, hydration. Can add Dantrolene + Dopamine agonist (Amantadine).
      d. Risk Factor – *Lewy Body Dementia* (alpha synuclein is the marker) = very much at risk for NMS!

438. Serotonin Syndrome – hyperreflexia and myoclonus

439. Don't prescribe benzodiazepine's to old folks! → At risk for confusion, falls, agitation

440. Cc: Sudden onset psychosis in a *child*? → Rule out SLE

441. Side effect of abrupt discontinuation of benzodiazepine (esp. Alprazolam)?
    a. Seizure

442. Euthyroid Sick Syndrome
    a. Seen in calorie restricted or ICU patients
    b. Thyroid hormone levels → low T3, normal T4 & TSH
    c. Dx: Elevated Reverse T3. Exclude hypothyroidism
    d. Rx: Treat the underlying nonthyroidal systemic illness

443. Idiopathic Thrombocytopenic Purpura (ITP)
    a. *No splenomegaly*
    b. Elevated megakaryocytes
    c. History of viral illness (URI)
    d. Associated with lymphoma, CLL, HIV, connective tissue diseases
    e. Chronic and insidious course with adults
    f. Rx: IV Immunoglobulin (IVIG), Steroids, Prednisone, Splenectomy
        i. Ddx → Rx for TTP and HUS is Plasmapheresis

444. Alkaline Phosphatase (ALP) – Made by liver and bone

445. Gamma-Glutamyl Transferase (GGT) – Made by liver only
    a. Alcohol raises GGT = marker for alcoholism
    b. GGT greatly elevated in obstructive jaundice, alcoholic liver disease, and hepatic cancer.

446. Gout – negative birefringence, needle-shaped monosodium urate crystals, *elevated wbc*

447. Immune insults like chemotherapy predispose to varicella zoster flares

448. Transillumination of a painless scrotal mass indicates a hydrocele, which is due to a patent process vaginalis.

449. DVT leads to erythema and venous engorgement

450. Mycoplasma pneumonia is treated with macrolide (erythromycin, clarithromycin)

451. Rx for gram negative rods (like E. coli) in a pregnant woman?
    a. Amoxicillin or Nitrofurantoin

452. Mother of twins is at increased risk for pre-term labor and delivery, HTN, pre-eclampsia, and intrahepatic cholestasis of pregnancy.

453. "Intracellular inclusion bodies" = CMV infection

454. Irritable Bowel Syndrome (IBS)
    a. Pain relieved by defecation
    b. Symptoms: chronic diarrhea, lower abdominal pain
    c. Rx: TCA (ex: Nortriptyline)

455. How to treat a hypertensive crisis caused by ingesting a tyramine rich food while on a MAO-I?
    a. Phentolamine (alpha blocker) or Nifedipine (calcium channel blocker)

456. Rx for catatonia?
    a. Benzodiazepine (lorazepam)

457. Se of Lithium?
    a. Seizure, nystagmus, confusion, AV block, hypothyroidism

458. Acute rx for adjustment disorder or suicidality after a stressor?
    a. Lorazepam or buspirone

459. Simple partial seizures have <u>no</u> loss of consciousness, aura, or déjà vu

460. Loss of consciousness in a seizure:
    a. Partial seizure with secondary generalization
        i. Tonic-clonic activity
        ii. Loss of bladder or bowel control, tongue biting
    b. Complex partial seizure
        i. +Motor automatisms (chewing, lip smacking, sucking)
        ii. Aura, bilateral motor findings sometimes

461. "To and Fro" murmur aka continuous machinery murmur?
    a. Patent Ductus Arteriosus (PDA)
    b. Wide pulse pressure with bounding peripheral pulses
    c. Recurrent lower respiratory tract infections
    d. Lower extremity clubbing
    e. CHF

462. Hyaline casts
    a. Cylindrical, clear casts
    b. Secreted by nephrons during *dehydration* and vigorous exercise
    c. Indicates low flow, acidic environment, concentrated urine

463. Hemothorax = blood in the pleural space
    a. Dx: Xray shows <u>blunting</u> of the costophrenic angle or <u>opacification</u> of the hemithorax
    b. Decreased or absent breath sounds on affected side
    c. Dull resonance on percussion

      d. Narrow pulse pressure
      e. Tachycardia, hypotension
      f. Rx: Chest tube (thoracostomy) at 6th or 7th intercostal space, midaxillary line

464. Testicular problems
    a. Varicocele
        i. Dilated pampiniform venous plexus of spermatic cord= "bag of worms"
        ii. Changes size when you lie down (it goes away).
        iii. Rx: Surgery
    b. Hydrocele
        i. Fluid accumulation within the tunica vaginalis. Transilluminates
        ii. Rx: Surgery
    c. Spermatocele
        i. Painless, cystic mass at the head of the epididymis that transilluminates
        ii. Rx: None, resolves on its own

465. Myelomeningocele can lead to Arnold-Chiari malformation = hydrocephalus due to obstruction of CSF outflow.

466. Hypercalcemia symptoms mimic Diabetes Mellitus symptoms! Calcium messes up ADH sensitivity.

467. Lumbar spinal stenosis → associated with osteoarthritis
    a. Cc: old guy with back pain while walking
    b. Pain <u>radiates</u> into buttocks and thighs bilaterally
    c. Pain worse when walking downhill
    d. Ankle-Brachial Index (ABI) is normal
    e. Pain relieved by leaning forward
    f. Dx: MRI
    g. Rx: NSAID or surgery

468. Vertebral Compression Fracture
    a. Acute back pain and <u>point tenderness</u> after strenuous activity
    b. Lying on back makes the pain less intense
    c. Pain does not radiate
    d. Decreased spinal mobility after bending, <u>coughing</u>, or lifting
    e. Pain not relieved by rest
    f. Caused by osteoporosis, osteomyelitis, hyperparathyroidism, Paget's Disease
    g. Hyperkyphosis is a complication
    h. Rx: Back brace + NSAID

469. Cervical Spondylosis (Osteoarthritis)
    a. Age related wear and tear of spinal column leading to <u>nerve root</u> compression
    b. Chronic <u>neck pain</u>, numbness in arms, limited neck rotation
    c. Dx: Xray shows osteophytes, narrowing of disc spaces, sclerotic facets
    d. <u>Hypertrophic</u> vertebral bodies

e. Rx: NSAID

470. Spondylolisthesis (Slipped disc)
    a. Forward displacement of a vertebral disc in relation to spine
    b. Stiff back, leaning-forward helps posture, "waddle" gait, atrophy of gluteal muscles.
    c. Generalized lower back pain, with intermittent shooting pain from buttocks to posterior thigh via sciatic nerve.
    d. Sitting and trying to stand up may be painful. Coughing and sneezing intensify pain.
    e. Dx: Xray of lower spine
    f. Rx: Nonsurgical rx first (back brace, physical therapy, NSAID). Spinal fusion surgery if nonsurgical rx does not work.

471. Cc: Old folks on "tea and toast" diet, bleeding gums? → Vitamin C deficiency

472. Epidural anesthesia in a pregnant woman can cause complication of *maternal hypotension*.

473. Before asymptomatic pts with diabetes mellitus, men older than 45, and women older than 55 start a vigorous new exercise regimen, they should undergo exercise treadmill testing.

474. Rapid strep test (to detect bacterial pharyngitis caused by group A streptococci) has a high false positive (FP) rate. It can only "rule in", so if negative still need to do throat culture!

475. EBV is the one virus that presents with an exudate.

476. Mitral Stenosis leads to pulmonary hypertension

477. Huntington's Disease – Seen in pts 40+ years old
    a. Chorea (vermicular movements of tongue + writhing movements)
    b. Memory loss
    c. Personality changes + psychosis

478. TB can have hilar adenopathy + pleural effusion

479. Aspergillus can also cause hilar adenopathy, but you need the pt. to have a prior history of asthma. Eosinophilia will be seen.

480. Transudate has < 3.0 g/dL protein. Transudate has > 59 mg/dL glucose.

481. Bone Marrow suppression leading to neutropenic fever is another side effect of carbamazepine and phenytoin.

482. Intraductal papilloma of breast
    a. Seen in perimenopausal women
    b. Spontaneous *bloody* discharge from one breast
    c. Dx: Mammogram, duct sonography to confirm
    d. Rx: Excisional biopsy

483. Ventricular Septal Defect (VSD) = Holosystolic murmur along left lower sternal border
    a. Cc: An infant with a large VSD will fail to thrive and become sweaty with feeds and tachypneic. The pulmonary vascular resistance will be high early on (until the VSD closes) so you won't hear the murmur early on nor have symptoms.

484. Treat acute transplant rejections by increasing the corticosteroid dose

485. ACE-I slow the progression of diabetic nephropathy

486. Lead poisoning
    a. Memory loss
    b. Interstitial nephritis
    c. Microcytic anemia with basophilic stippling
    d. Wrist drop, foot drop

487. Empyema = pus in the pleural space. Is a complication of pneumonia. Think of it as a pleural effusion that gets infected.

488. Complex Partial Seizure (Temporal Lobe Seizure)
    a. Arises in one lobe of the brain, rather than the whole brain
    b. Most common type of seizure experienced by people with epilepsy
    c. Briefly lose contact with reality
    d. Series of autonomic gestures: Lip smacking, picking at clothing, hand wringing
    e. Can smell burning rubber

489. Malignant HTN Rx?
    a. Nitroprusside, IV Labetalol

490. Triglyceride-induced pancreatitis → Look for triglyceride levels 1000-2000

491. Acute rx for gout?
    a. Indomethacin (NSAID), Colchicine, Steroids (glucocorticoids)

492. Magnesium Sulfate cannot be given to women with Myasthenia Gravis!
    a. Nifedipine (Ca channel blocker) is now used to prevent premature labor
    b. Terbutaline (Beta2 agonist) now is not used because se of cardiac arrhythmias

493. Hyper IgE (Job's) Syndrome
    a. Defective STAT3 signaling protein leads to defective Th17 cells. This leads to impaired recruitment of neutrophils.

494. Ataxia-Telangiectasia – poor smooth pursuit of moving target with eyes
    a. Dx: Elevated AFP

495. Leukocyte Adhesion Deficiency (LAD)
    a. Defective neutrophil adhesion leads to neutrophilia and inability to form pus
    b. Integrin CD18 is defective
    c. Recurrent bacterial infections beginning in the neonatal period
    d. Cc: Child with severe oral pain due to gingivitis

496. Baby with PCP Pneumonia?
    a. Hyper IgM Syndrome
    b. Di George Syndrome

497. Cancerous lesion observed in the lips
    a. Upper lip = basal cell carcinoma
    b. Lower lip = squamous cell carcinoma

498. Thalassemia → Mentzer Index (MCV/RBC) < 13
    a. Iron deficiency anemia → Mentzer Index > 13

499. Polycystic Ovarian Syndrome (PCOS)
    a. Elevated LH → Elevated Testosterone
    b. Decreased FSH → Decreased Progesterone (unopposed estrogen!)
        i. 17apha-OH deficiency

500. Stroke in a *young* person?
    a. Polyarteritis Nodosa

501. Oxycodone abuse leads to euphoria, joy, release of muscle tension
    a. Se: constipation, nausea & vomiting (n/v), confusion, pinpoint pupils
    b. Withdrawal signs: n/v, diarrhea, anxiety, shaking, coughing

502. Drug to use for alcohol withdrawal?
    a. Acamprosate

503. Buprenorphine
    a. For rx of opioid addiction
    b. Partial agonist, so no risk of respiratory depression, unlike methadone

504. Post-Op Fever. Remember the order with this mnemonic. Think about a hurricane:
    a. First, the Wind then the Rain (Water) then you run (Walk) then you trip and fall (Wound), and you Wonder what happened to get the abscess
    b. Now just add the day it presents with ascending odd numbers 1 3 5 7 + 10 for abscess.

505. Agoraphobia

      a. Rx: Exposure therapy

506. Social Anxiety Disorder
    a. Rx: SSRI, Beta blocker for performance situations (ex: giving a speech)

507. DVT in pregnancy
    a. Dx: Venous compression doppler ultrasound
    b. Rx: Heparin (LMWH)

508. Cc: Man in Montana contracted West Nile virus. How to prevent?
    a. Wear long-sleeved shirts

509. Toluene (paint thinner) toxicity
    a. Toxicity symptoms: euphoria, *hallucinations*, seizures, dizziness, ataxia, anion-gap metabolic acidosis.
    b. Withdrawal symptoms: nausea, irritability, tremor, agitation, dry mouth

510. Legg-Calve-Perthes disease = avascular necrosis of the femoral head

511. Chronic Lymphocytic Leukemia (CLL)
    a. Abnormal proliferation of B lymphocytes, and they are clonal, either kappa or lambda.
    b. Smudge cells
    c. Confirm via flow cytometry for CD5+, CD20+

512. Rx for Lung Cancer
    a. Small cell → chemotherapy
    b. Squamous cell → Resect, follow up with radiation and chemotherapy

513. Hydrops Fetalis is due to fetal anemia

514. Bartonella henselae (cat scratch disease) is rx with azithromycin or doxycycline

515. Pasteurella multocida (cat bite disease) is rx with amoxicillin-clavulanate
    a. Rx requires both aerobic and anaerobic coverage

516. How to confirm Addison's disease?
    a. Cosyntropin test

517. What vaccine cannot be given to a pregnant woman?
    a. Varicella zoster vaccine

518. Remember that MMR and Influenza vaccines can be given to person with egg allergy

519. CIWA protocol is indicating moderate alcohol withdrawal, what is the next step?

a. Give Diazepam 20 mg q.1-2 hours until symptoms become mild

520. Woman is newly diagnosed with Bartholin cyst, what is the next step?
    a. I & D (catheterization)

521. Triceps reflex = C7

522. Laryngomalacia = stridor worse in supine position and improves in prone position. GERD is a comorbid condition.

523. Bladder cancer risk factors?
    a. Smoking is the #1 risk factor
    b. Occupational risk factors: painter, truck driver, hair dresser
    c. Drug use risk factor: pioglitazone

524. Diffusion Capacity (DLCO)
    a. Decreased in both restrictive diseases and obstructive disease (emphysema only)
    b. DLCO is normal in chronic bronchitis
    c. DLCO is elevated in asthma

525. Myotonic muscular dystrophy
    a. Cc: Man can't release hand grip
    b. Baldness, testicular atrophy, cataracts

526. +Babinski (plantar extension) sign = lesion at corticospinals (pyramidal sign)

527. +Romberg sign = dorsal column lesion

Congratulations! You have reached the end. I hope this book has proven useful to you as you prepare for the USMLE Step 2 CK Exam. One final piece of advice: do the sample test questions aka "The Free 120" on the Usmle.org website. My students have told me that they have seen verbatim repeat questions on the actual exam! I sincerely wish you all the best in your journey towards medical residency. – John Thomas, MD

About the Author

Dr. John Thomas, MD is an independent medical researcher whose main area of interest is nutrition.

www.ingramcontent.com/pod-product-compliance
Lightning Source LLC
Chambersburg PA
CBHW080955220526
45465CB00008BA/3293